HOW TO CURE HPV WARTS FOR GOOD

Pamphlet

By N.A.R

PREFACE

A lot of people have HPV or genital warts and are scared to let anyone know because of the stigmatism behind having a sexually transmitted infection. Some warts are not sexually transmitted so please do a research on the type of wart you have and its proper treatment. These set of instructions are to help you remove the wart and stop them from coming back for good. According to the CDC 90% or warts are caused by HPV 6 or 11. I am a nurse and I have applied this technique before with excellent results. This is for people who have tried all the treatments at their doctor's office or at home and still can't get rid of these pesky little things that itches, embarrass and annoy them daily.

WHAT ARE WARTS?

Warts are small raised skin surfaces in a tiny dot or cauliflower shape. They can be rough and sometimes flat like little tine plaques of skin. They can be transferred by touch so during this treatment please abstain from any sexual contact and also make sure your partner gets treated as well. There are other treatments that you can try but they normally result with the warts coming back. A few such treatments are with a drug called Podofilox, Sinecatechin a green tea extract or cryotherapy. There is no guarantee that removing the warts will cure the HPV virus. The warts are just a manifestation of the virus in the upper layer of the skin.

WARNING!

WHAT YOU WILL NEED

For this treatment you will need a few items. These are not hard to get items because you can pick them up at your local grocery store. You will need some swabs or Q-tips as they are commonly known as, a small bowl, cayenne pepper, a safety pin or needle, baking soda, vitamin E oil, lemon juice and some aloe Vera juice. If the warts are around your anus area you might need a handheld mirror and a flashlight, or you can use the flashlight on your phone.

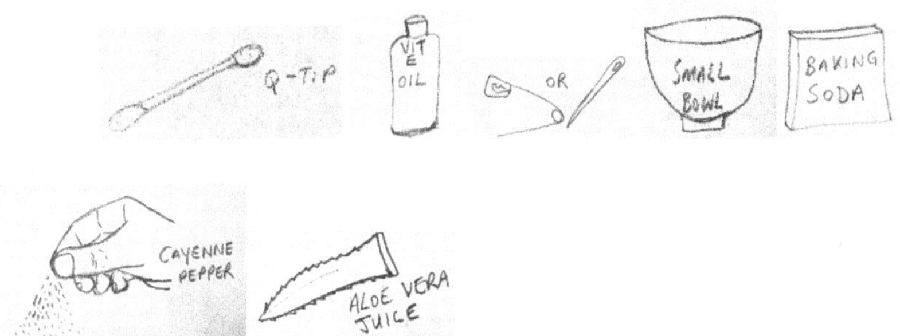

Add the following ingredients to the small bowl and mix together into a paste:

1 tablespoon baking soda

1 tablespoon vitamin E oil

1 small pinch of cayenne pepper

2 tablespoons aloe Vera juice

1 tablespoon lemon juice

After adding the ingredients together clean the area where the warts are with soap and water and also make sure the needle or safety pin is wipe thoroughly with alcohol. If you are not sure then place the needle and or safety pin in a small container with alcohol and then clean them off with a clean napkin after every use. The reason for this is because you are going to be pricking or sticking the wart with the needles to irritate and break the skin on the wart, so the ointment can penetrate and destroy the blood vessels that supplies the wart with nutrients.

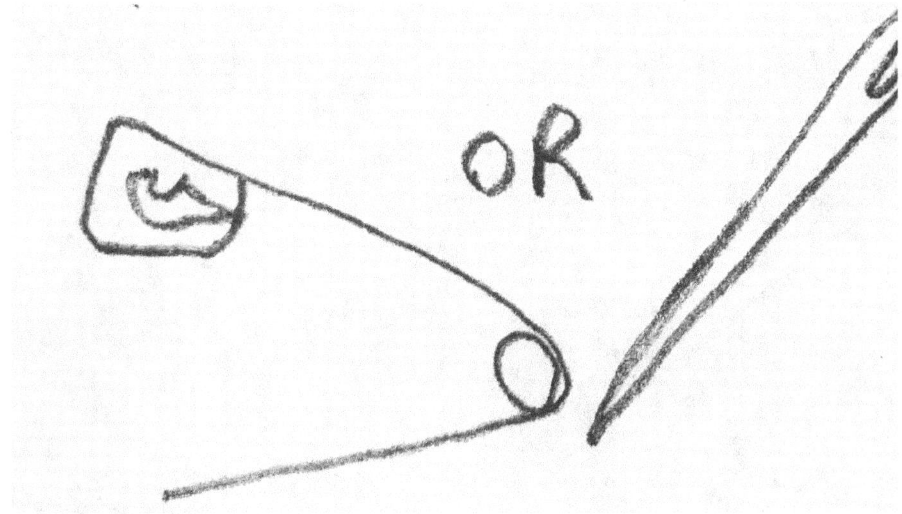

Take the safety pin and gently break or prick the wart. A little bit or blood might weep or seep out of the wart. Do not panic. If you are on blood thinners or any medication that thins the blood, please do not attempt this and let your doctor know before you attempt doing this. If you are not good at standing pain because of heart problems or other mental or physical problems relating to a bad reaction to pain or any allergic reaction to any of the ingredients, please do not try this.

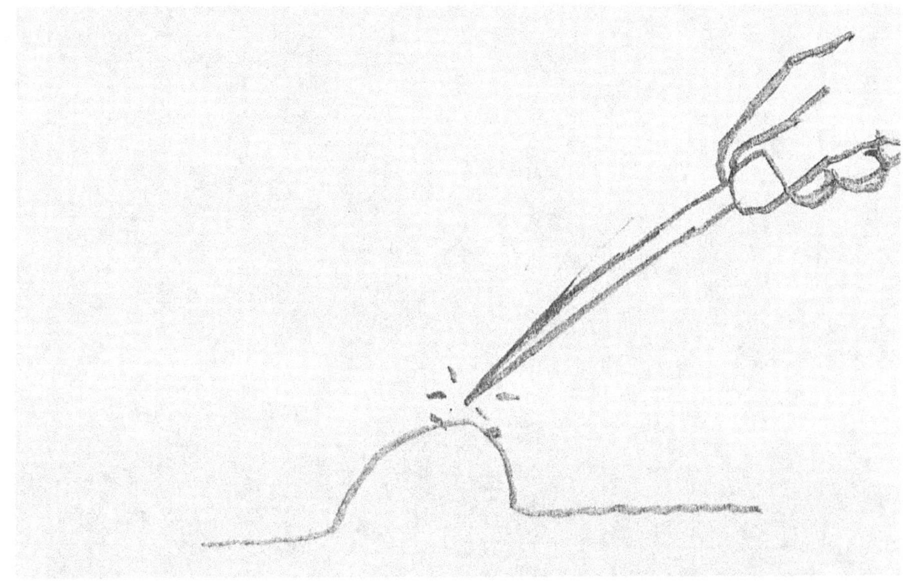

Use the swab or Q-tip to apply the ointment directly to the wart. A few dabs should be good. If the warts are around the anal area, please do not touch the tip to the anal opening because this will burn you for a long time. Please remember this procedure is painful as described above in the warning page of the book. The ointment will burn you as well when applied to the warts.

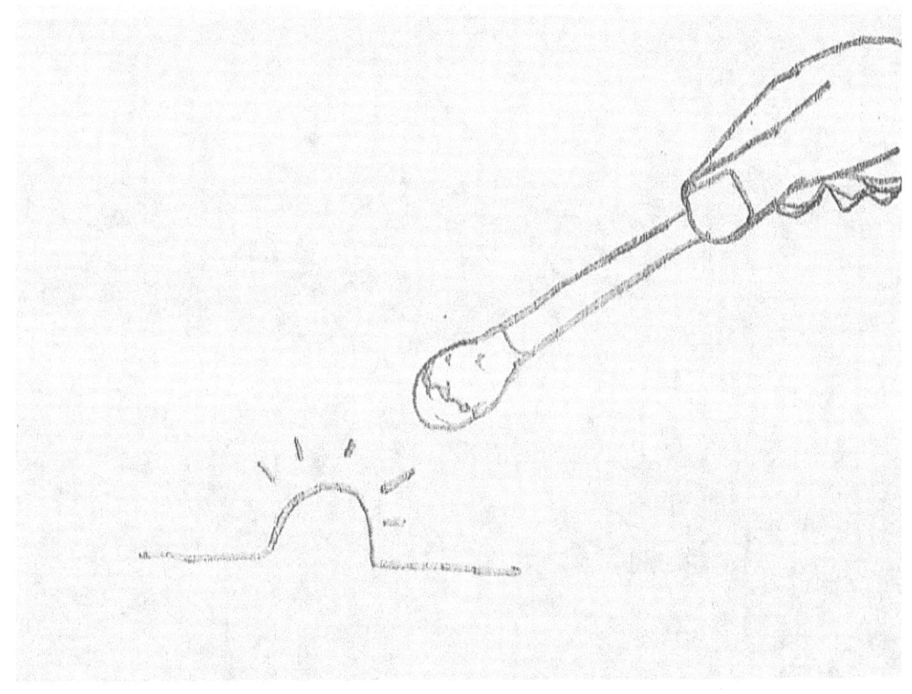

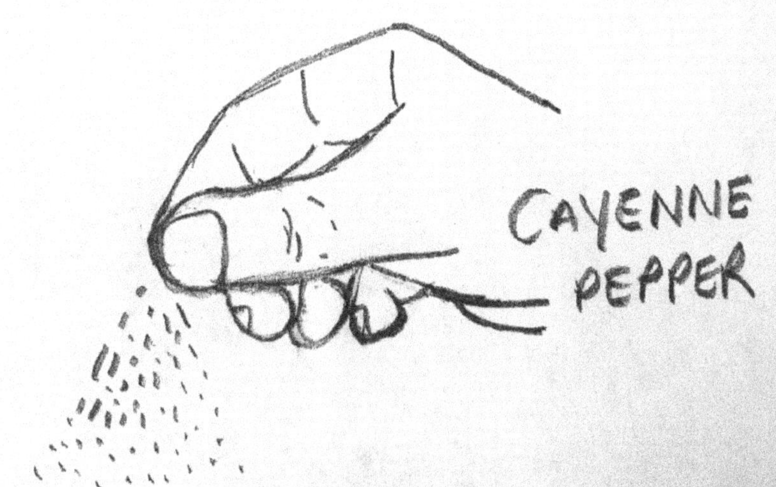
CAYENNE
PEPPER

If you are applying it to the inside of your buttock cheeks close to your anus, please remember to clean the area and all items before using them. You will need a small handheld mirror which you will place on a surface lower than you, preferably the floor, facing up so you can see your anus area. You will need a flashlight to illuminate the area as well. You can use the flashlight on your phone facing upwards to illuminate the area, so you can properly see what you are doing. Please do not perch on or climb on unsteady or unsafe surfaces to accomplish this. Please make sure you are physically capable of bending in a squatting position and being able to get back up. Prick the warts as stated above and apply ointment with the tip of a Q-tip.

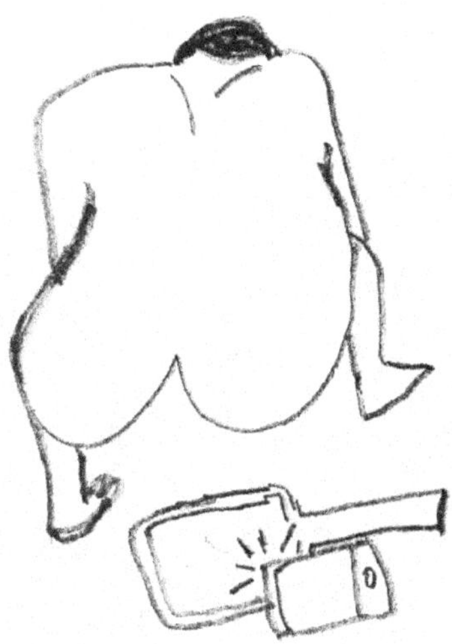

The good thing about warts is that they will not return in the same exact spot. They will return a few centimeters from where the last wart was destroyed. So, the more you destroy them the more they will run out of real-estate to flourish. In order for this to work you must apply it for up to four times a week and then let the warts die. They will return again in most cases and you can tell by the itchy feeling and raised skin you will feel in that area. If you are not sure take some soap in your hand while showering and run your hands where the warts normally are. The water and soap should enhance your ability to feel if there is any raised skin in that area. While doing that just go ahead and wash that area with your bare hands and soap. For this treatment to work you must be consistent. Every time they return for the next 2 months you must repeat the steps above. After about 3 or more months the warts should disappear for good. If not keep applying until they do not return anymore. This shouldn't take long because after while the warts should go away. You must be CONSISTENT, or it will not work.

It takes time to get rid of them as they keep coming back your body will finally send the message they are no longer welcomed.

S	M	T	W	T	F	S
		1	2	3	4	5
6	7	8	9	10	11	12
13	14	15	16	17	18	19
20	21	22	23	24	25	26
27	28	29	30	31		

The method behind the ointment is as follows. The aloe Vera is to protect and sooth your skin as well as it helps to heal. The aloe Vera will also give your skin a fighting chance as it improves the immunity and antioxidant delivered to the skin. The vitamin E oil contains the perfect vitamin to help fight the wart as vitamin E is also an antioxidant and it nourishes the skin. The vitamin E oil also provides a barrier to cut off oxygen to the wart. The baking soda also helps to create a barrier blocking the oxygen to the wart as well as dry out the wart, so it can die off more quickly. Pricking the wart with the needle or safely pin is to help the ointment penetrate more and become more effective. Also pricking it will agitate it and let your body knows it is an invader and the body will fight back and help destroy the offending wart. When you prick or agitate the wart you are basically snitching on the wart to your body. The lemon juice will also provide vitamin C which is acidic to burn the wart. Vitamin C is also an antioxidant and helps to strengthen the immunity of the skin around the wart and protect the wart from any infection. Please make sure the area where the warts are being kept dry at all times. Sometimes the warts spread from the genital to the anus area because of the use of the same rag. Try using different rags in to wash or dry separate areas of your body. Also cut out eating unhealthy foods so your body can develop an immunity to the warts.

Cut out eating red meat and junk foods and eat a cleaner leaner diet until the warts go away.

Here are some other means in which to fight the wart that might not be as painful as the method shown above. You can soak a cotton ball in some aloe Vera juice and tape it over the wart. This will soften the wart and help to destroy the wart. You can get the aloe Vera in its juice form at your local grocery store. Please get the raw one and not an aloe Vera drink that is processed for oral consumption. If not, then get the plant and use the gel between the skin. Rub the gel on the wart and cover the wart. The aloe Vera plant contains malic acid which will break down the wart without any pain.

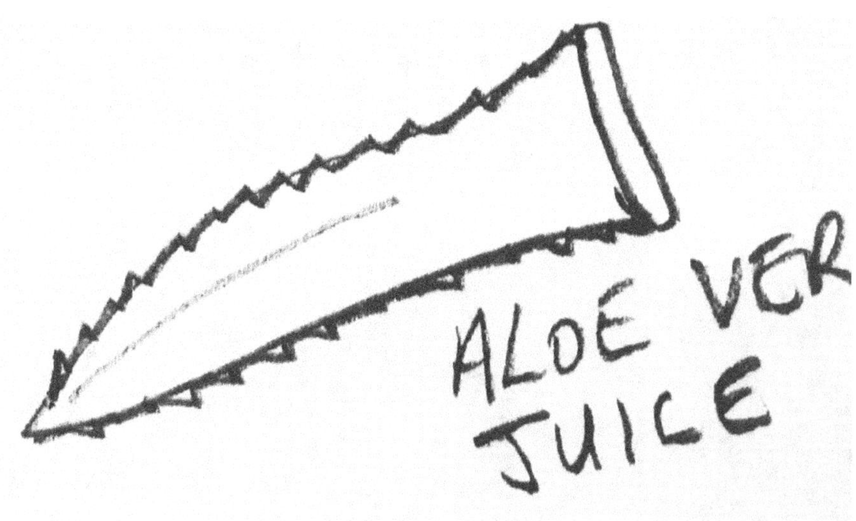

Another method is to use baking soda. You can mix castor oil with baking soda into a paste and apply it to the warts at nights. You can also crush up some basil and used it similarly or add it to the concoction of baking soda and castor oil. Baking soda is a strong anti-inflammatory that counteracts the virus causing the wart to form. The baking soda will break down the wart as the baking soda naturally exfoliate the skin cells that makes up the wart. It also causes a drying effect that dries out the wart and robs it of its moisture. You can also add a tablespoon of apple cider vinegar to make a paste with the baking soda to apply directly to the wart.

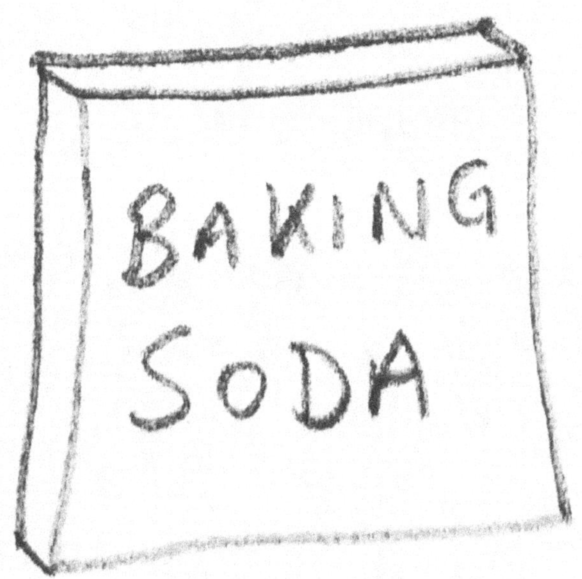

Also try aspirin and lemon juice. Add 2 aspirin tablets and 2 tablespoons of crushed aspirin into a paste. Apply directly to the wart. My best advice before applying anything to warts is to take a needle and prick the surface so that the ointment can penetrate and become more effective. Do not break the skin to cause excessive bleeding. Just scratch the surface as much as you can tolerate and apply the paste to the warts. Please remember in order to get results you must give the treatment time to work and follow up with more treatment as much as you can.

S	M	T	W	T	F	S
		1	2	3	4	5
6	7	8	9	10	11	12
13	14	15	16	17	18	19
20	21	22	23	24	25	26
27	28	29	30	31		

Here are also a few more combinations to use when fighting warts if you do not want to use the above treatment with the cayenne pepper. You can try mixing garlic and water to make a paste. Mix vitamin C tablets with water to make a paste. Break vitamin E capsules open and rub on the warts. Tea tree oil mixed with cloves or other oils such as frankincense oil. Applying pineapples freshly cut to the wart so that enzymes can destroy the wart is also a suggestion. Wash your hands and stop the spread as well as abstain from sexual or skin to skin contact until the warts go away. These methods might not be as effective as the warts will still return time and time again. But if you want to see results you might need to step up the heat and try the first method shown in the book. The only problem is it will irritate your skin as it will leave a burning effect for a few hours. Stick to it until the warts disappear for good. You will never get any lasting results if you give up after 2 months. The warts will die off and return in a different spot in the same area. The period it takes for them to die off and grow back can last up to two weeks. This is why it takes months to get rid of them permanently. Please remember to contact your professional healthcare provider before attempting anything stated in this book and get their professional advice. Do not try anything listed in this book if you are allergic to them or the ingredients when mixed together.